We Can Be Responsible!

WE STAY CLEAN

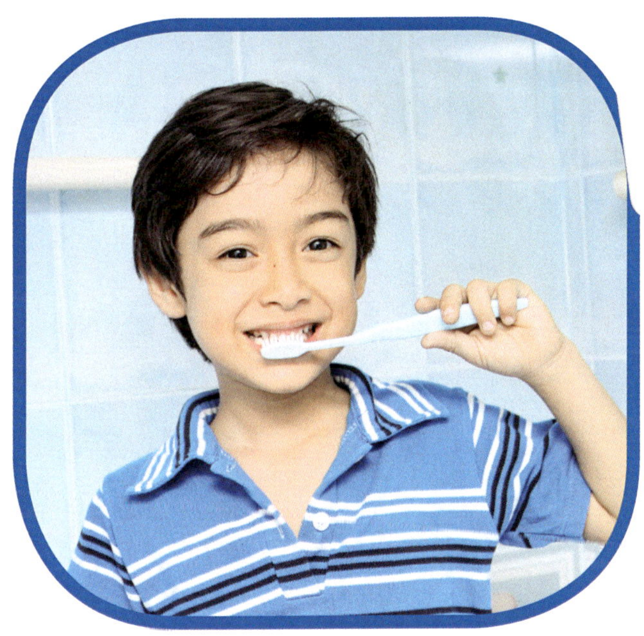

By Lynda Arnéz

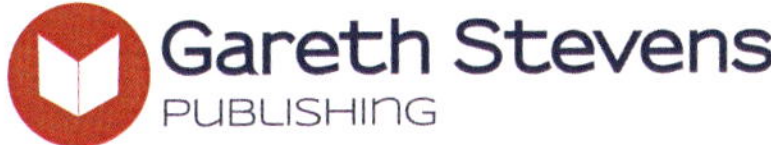

Please visit our website, www.garethstevens.com. For a free color catalog of all our high-quality books, call toll free 1-800-542-2595 or fax 1-877-542-2596.

Library of Congress Cataloging-in-Publication Data

Names: Arnéz, Lynda, author.
Title: We stay clean / Lynda Arnéz.
Description: New York : Gareth Stevens Publishing, [2020] | Series: We can be responsible! | Includes index.
Identifiers: LCCN 2018038759| ISBN 9781538239193 (pbk.) | ISBN 9781538239216 (library bound) | ISBN 9781538239209 (6 pack)
Subjects: LCSH: Hygiene–Juvenile literature.
Classification: LCC RA777 .A76 2020 | DDC 613–dc23
LC record available at https://lccn.loc.gov/2018038759

First Edition

Published in 2020 by
Gareth Stevens Publishing
111 East 14th Street, Suite 349
New York, NY 10003

Editor: Kristen Nelson
Designer: Sarah Liddell

Photo credits: Cover, p. 1 Littlekidmoment/Shutterstock.com; p. 5 didesign021/Shutterstock.com; p. 7 hanapon1002/Shutterstock.com; pp. 9, 24 (rubber duck) Amdezigns/Shutterstock.com; p. 11 Ermolaev Alexander/Shutterstock.com; pp. 13, 15, 24 (toothbrush) Raia/Shutterstock.com; p. 17 Anneka/Shutterstock.com; p. 19 Mr. Teerapong Kunkaeo/Shutterstock.com; p. 21 Africa Studio/Shutterstock.com; p. 23 XiXinXing/Shutterstock.com.

Printed in the United States of America

CPSIA compliance information: Batch #CS19GS: For further information contact Gareth Stevens, New York, New York at 1-800-542-2595.

Contents

Being clean is
part of staying healthy!

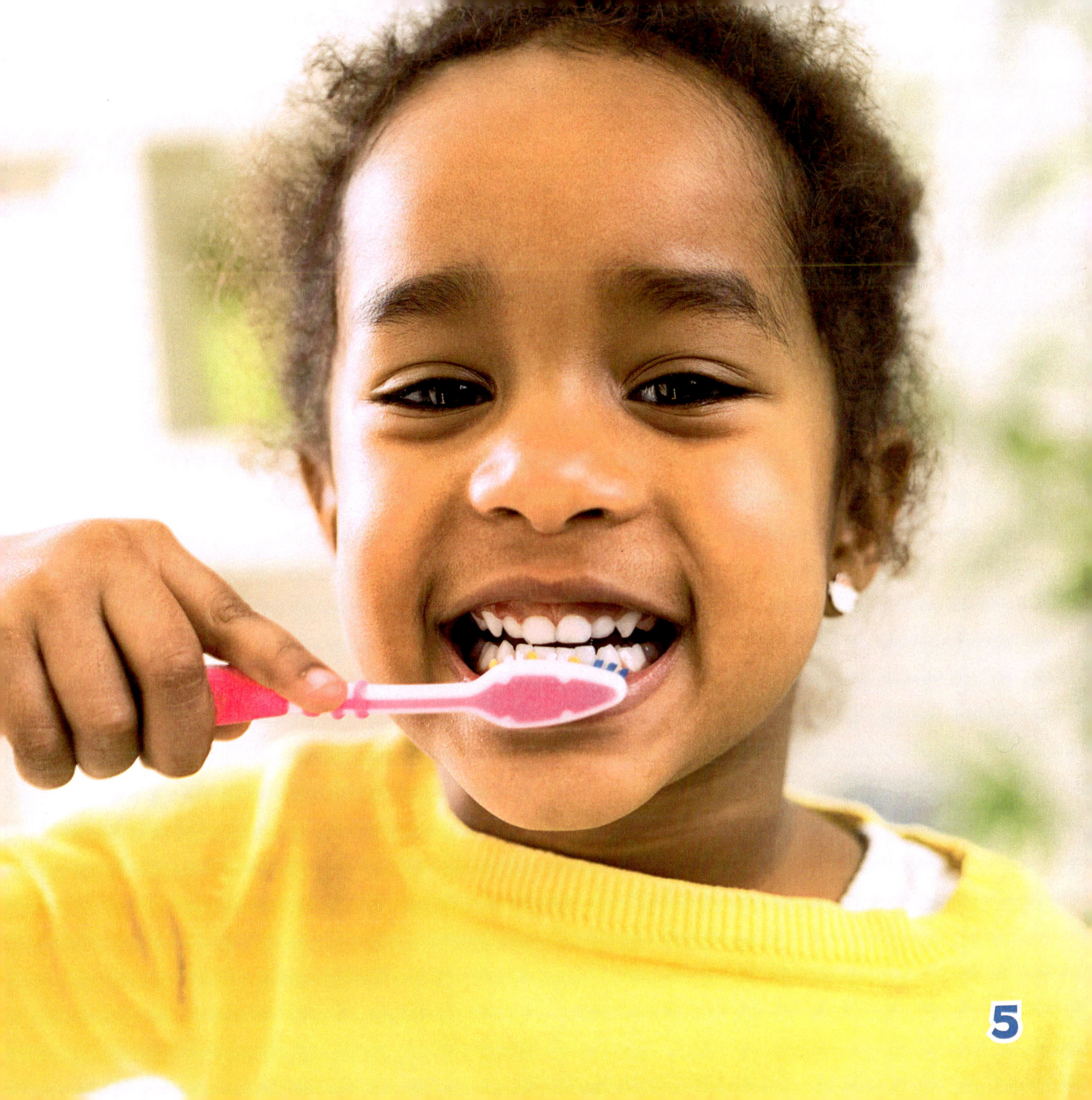

Kiara takes a bath
in the morning

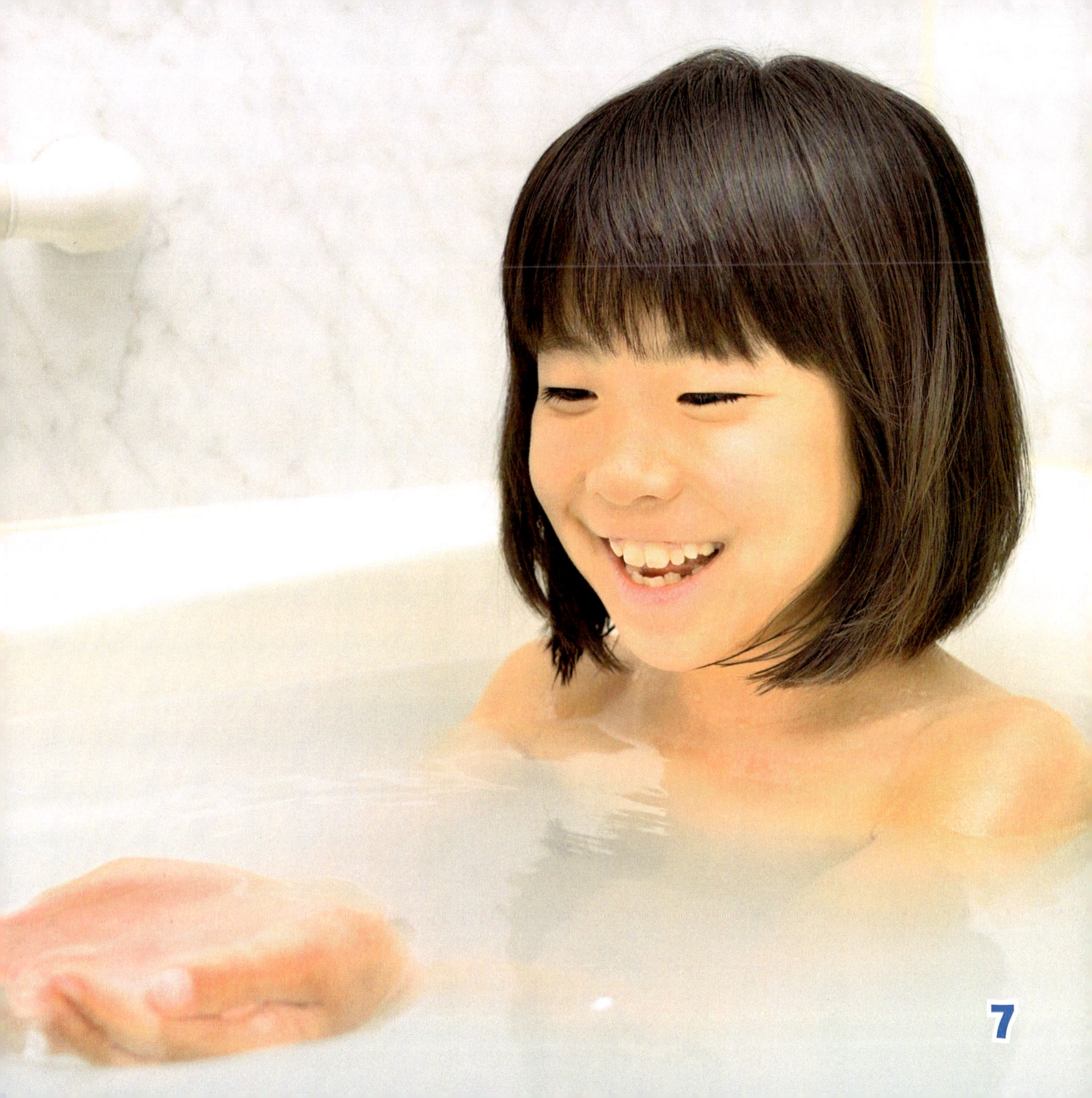

Gavin takes a bath
at night!
He plays with
rubber ducks.

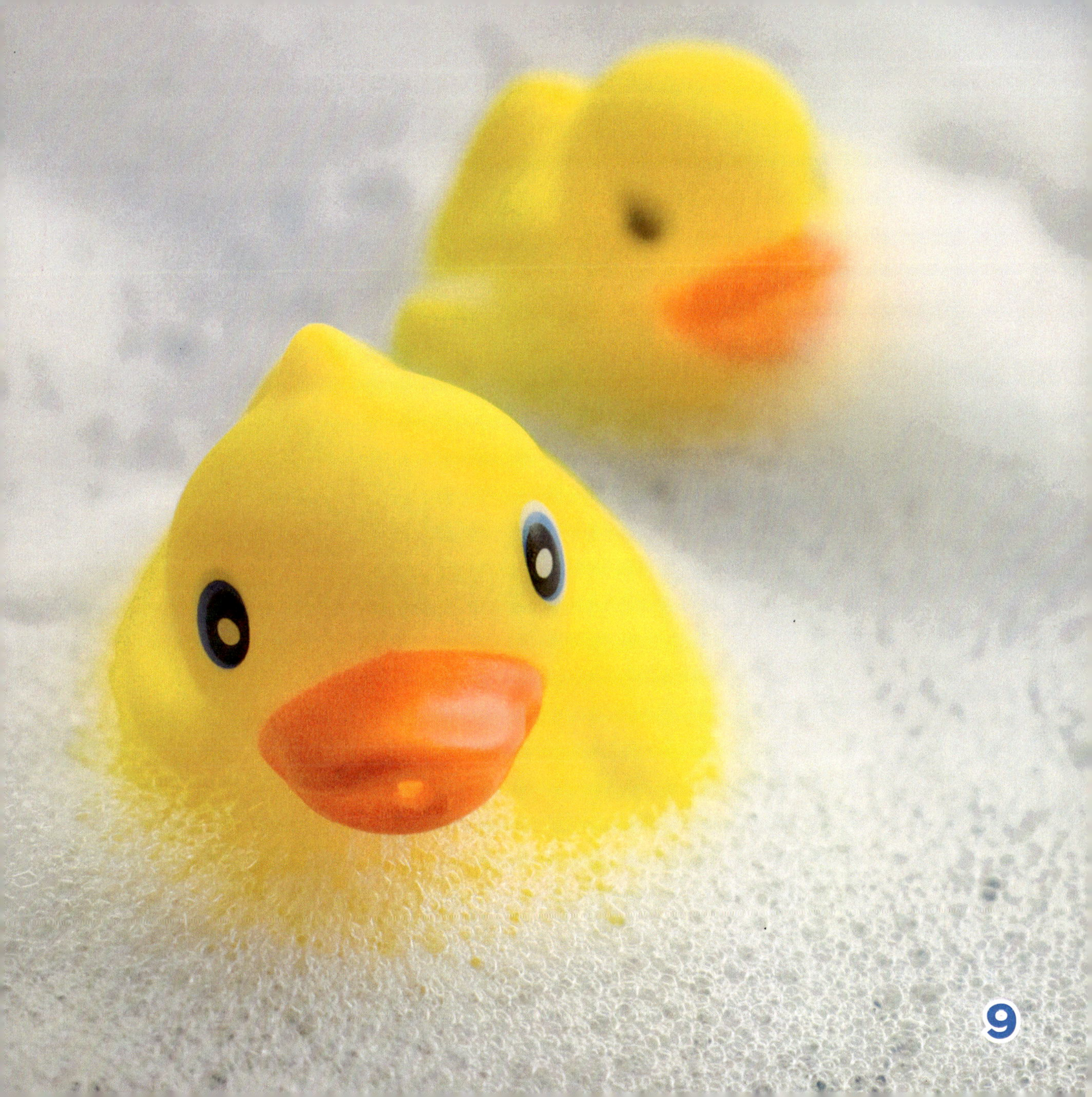

Zeke takes a shower.
He washes his hair.

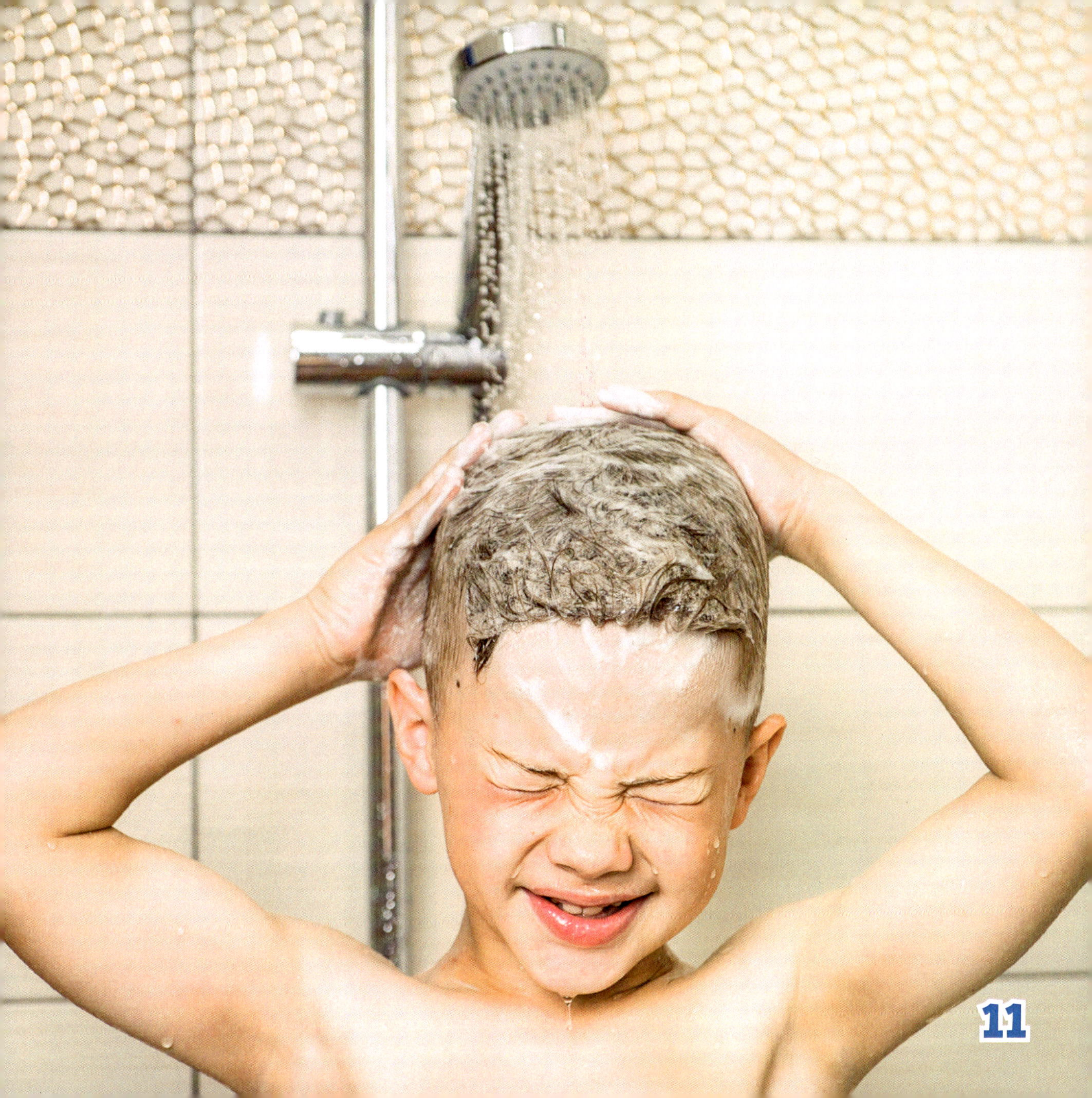

Delia washes her face.
She uses soap.

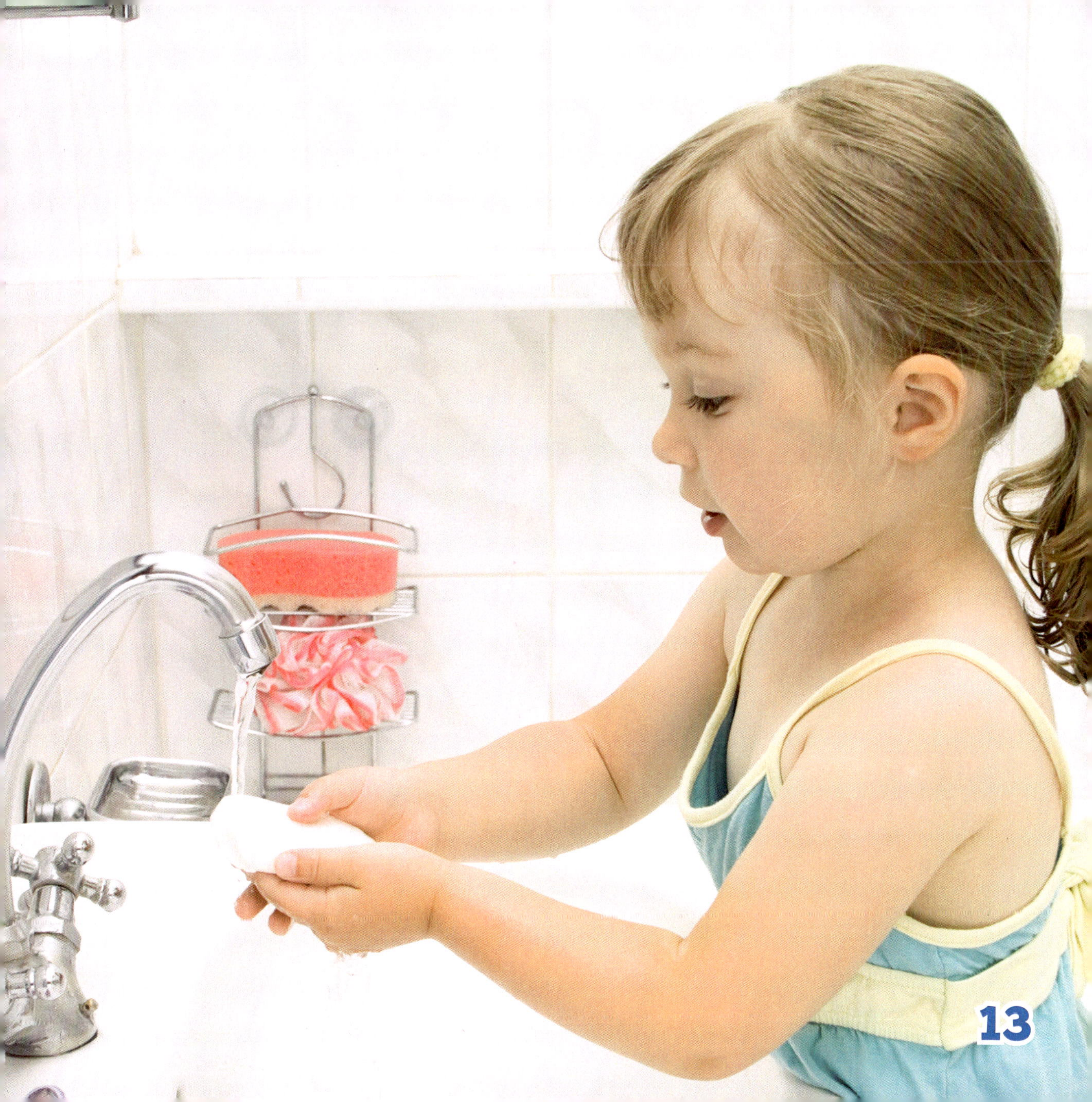

She keeps her teeth
clean, too.
She uses a toothbrush!

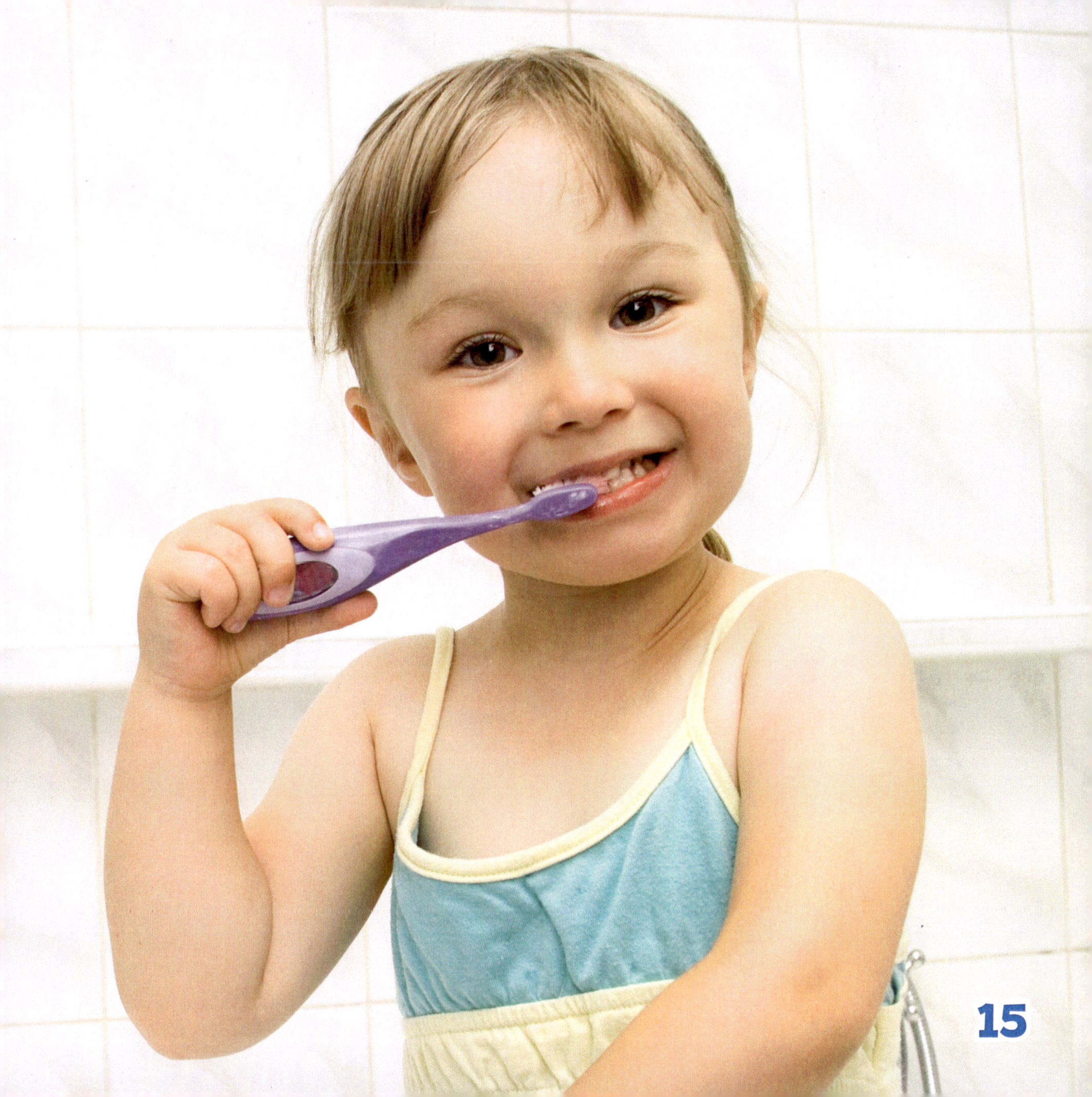

We got muddy
playing outside!
Time to clean up.

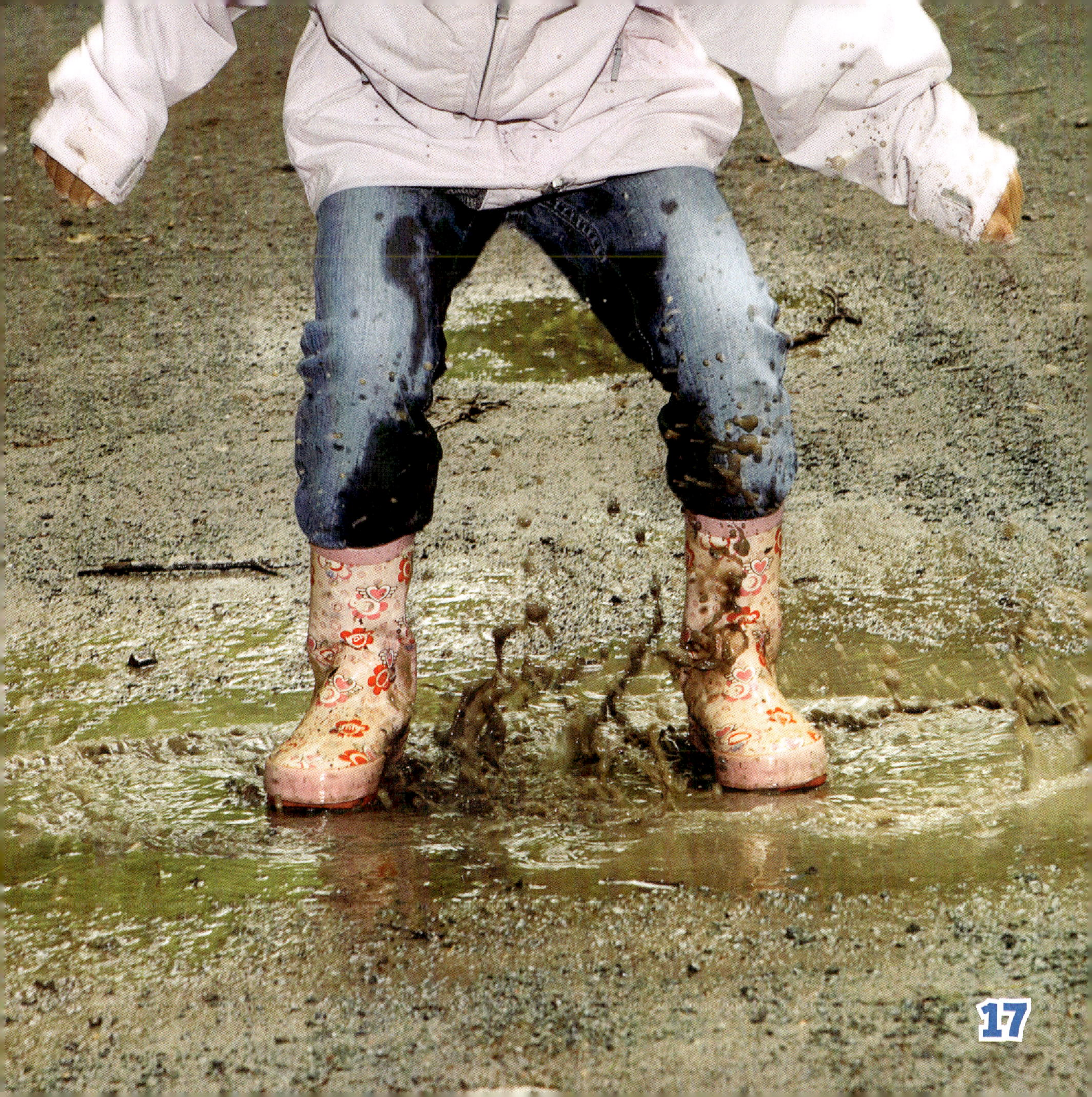

Erik washed between his toes!

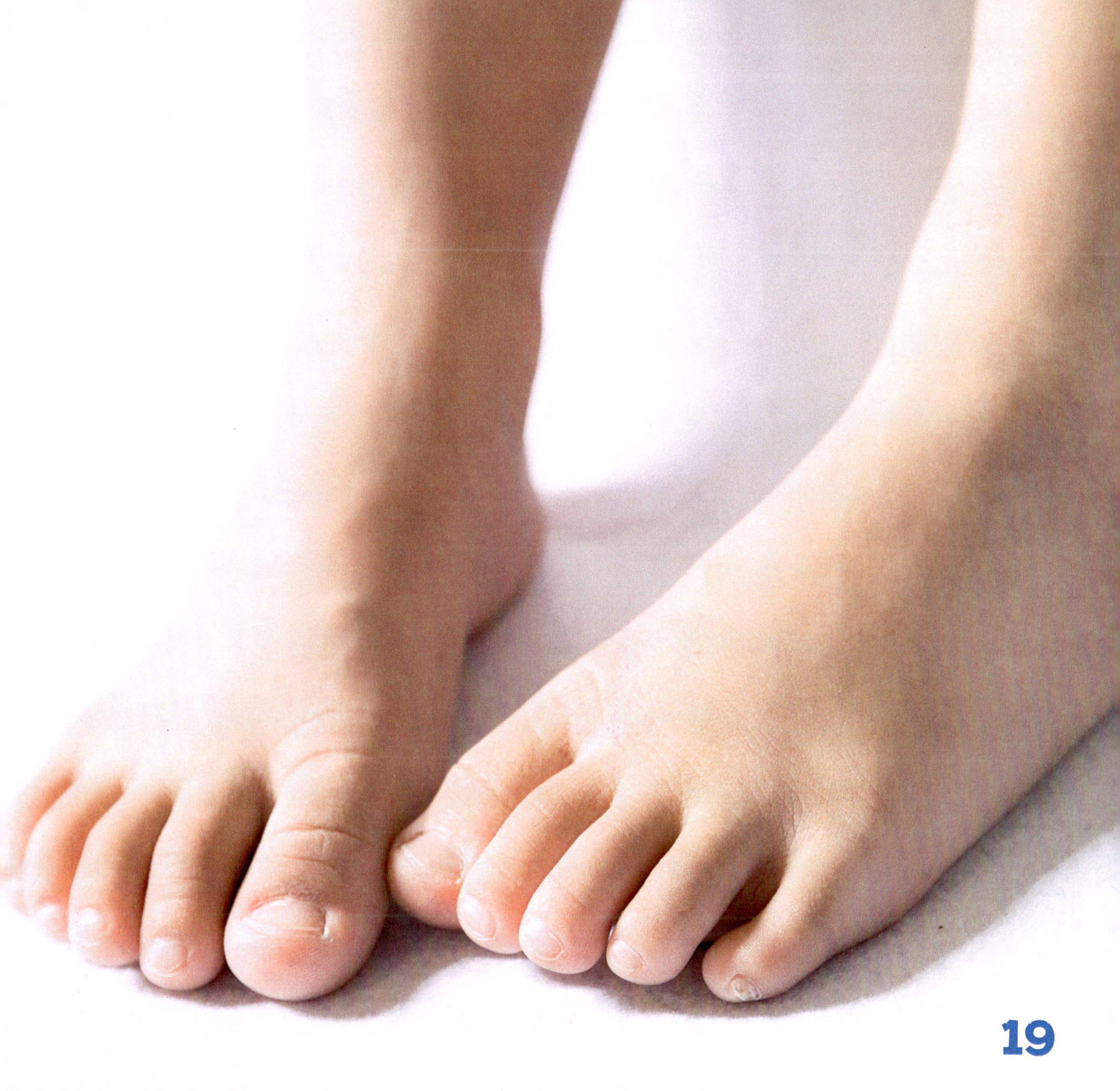

Lena washed her clothes.

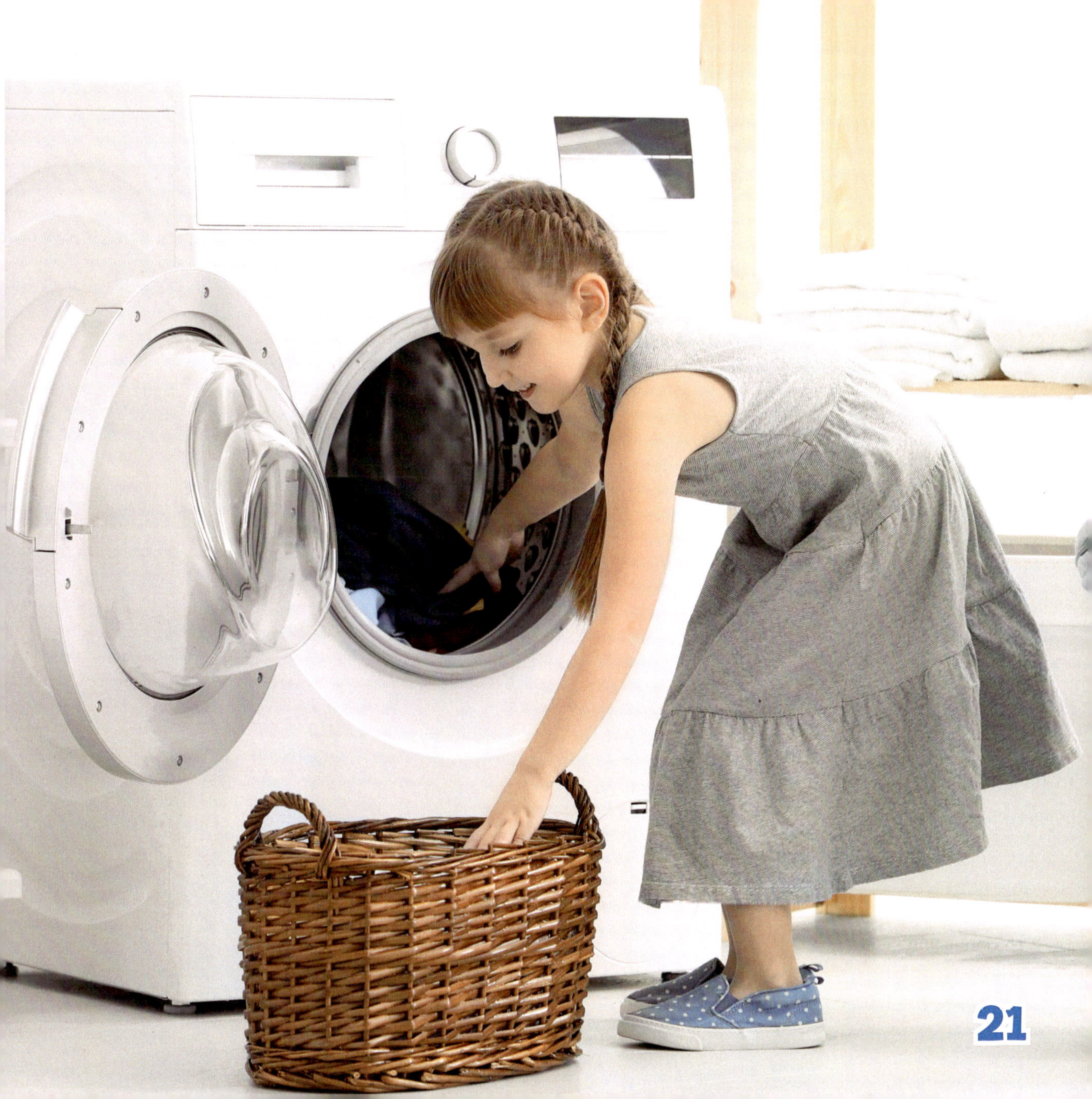

How do you stay clean?

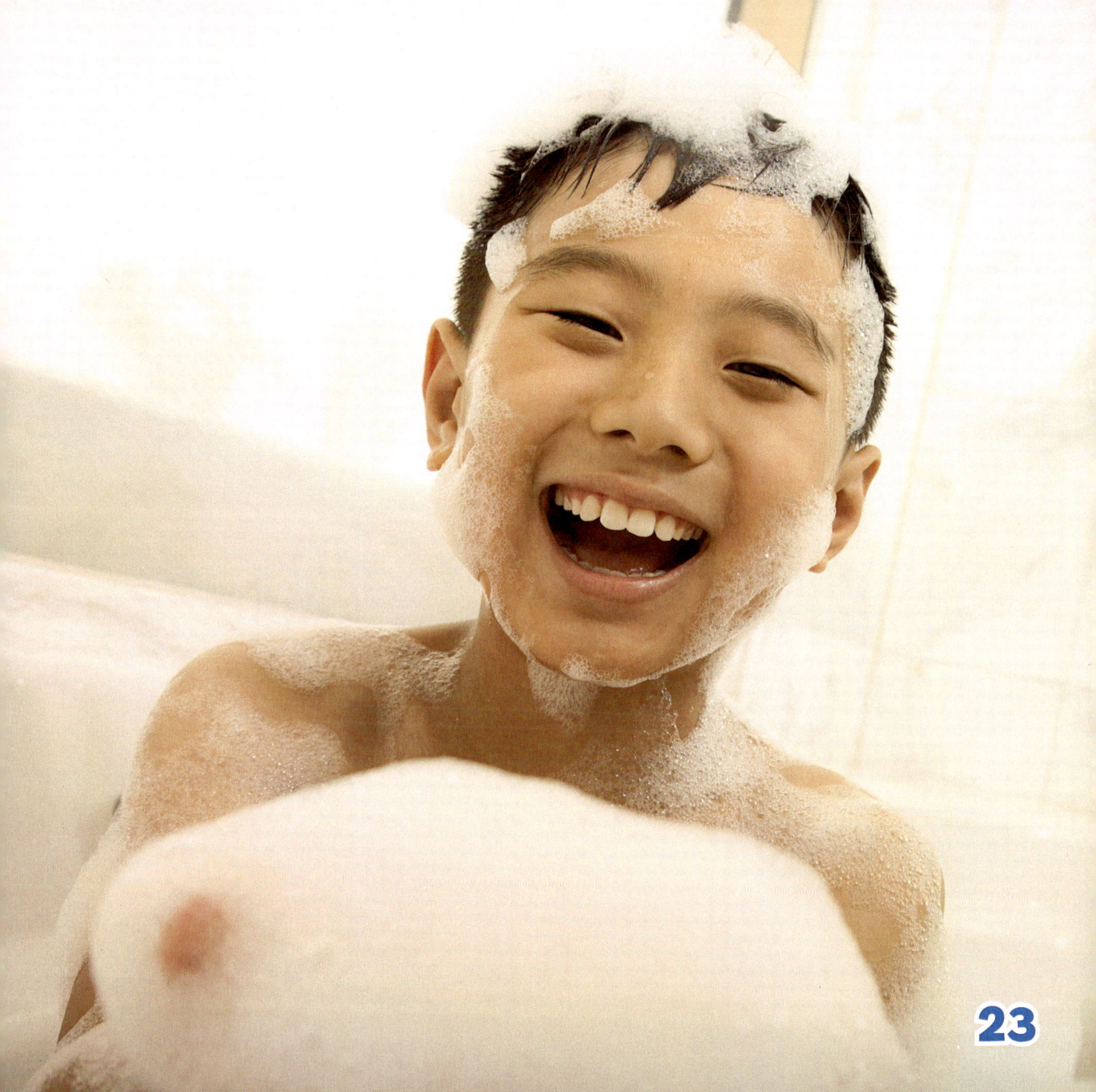

Words to Know

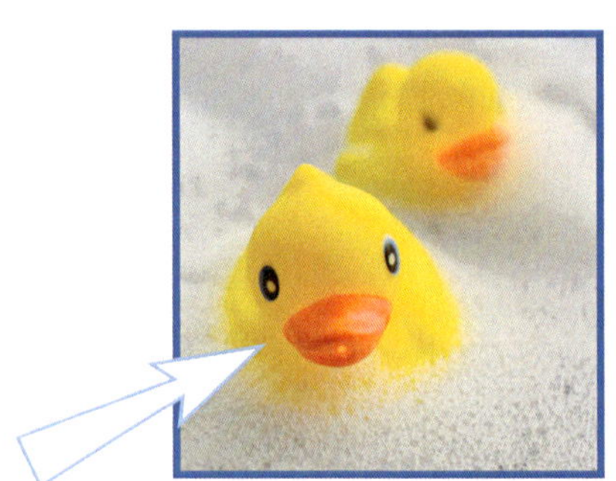

rubber duck

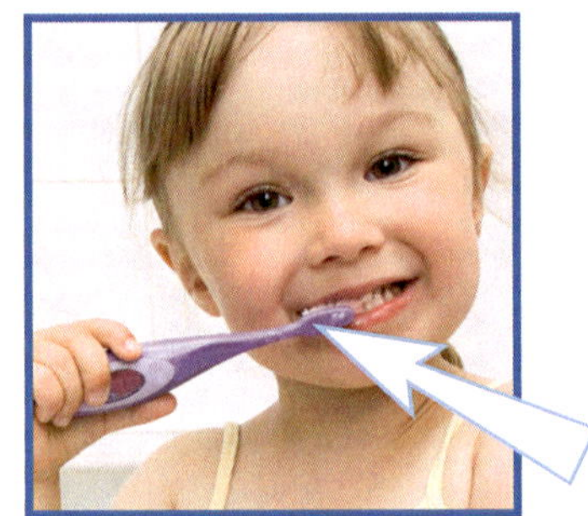

toothbrush

Index